Sex is NOT a Dirty Word

7 WAYS TO GET

COMFORTABLE

with your SEXUALITY

...with or without a partner

Jenifer Bartoszek

This book is intended to provide accurate and authoritative information in regard to the subject matter covered. It is sold with the understanding that the publisher is not engaged in rendering legal or other professional services. If legal advice or other expert assistance is required the services of a competent professional person should be sought.

Acknowledgements

I have had the great pleasure to meet and be inspired by some exceptional speakers and authors. Thank you Marcia Wieder, Jack Canfield, Caterina Rando, Tristan Taormino, Sam Horn and Jennifer Abernathy for your wisdom and expertise.

Heartfelt love and appreciation to my entire Athena's family, past, present, and future. You amaze me and motivate me to be the best I can be.

To my dream team, for you were there when it all started, sharing my dreams, believing in me and encouraging me every day. I treasure you.

For my dear friend and Mother Goddess, Jennifer Jolicoeur, for bringing all of these amazing people and endless opportunities into my life. You have shown me that everything is possible when you dream and when you believe, and I will be forever grateful.

Missy DeFrancesco Julian, Lynne Cumming, Dawn Brunt, Annie Dumas, Alessa Valles, James Thomas, Lauren Sembersky and the brilliant photographers who captured their sexy and allowed me to include them in this book.

Very special thanks to those who supported me and this release: Gina Ventullo, Nicole Vera, Amy Gray, Dylan Davis, Remy Tankel, Jason and Nicole Brown, Sharon Riley and Audrey Lambert.

Cheers to my friend Kristen Connolly, for inviting me to a party and introducing me to my destiny.

Many thanks to Rob and Tia Kelley for their friendship and patience as well as their collective creativity, talent, and innovation that truly made this a collaboration, and brought my vision to fruition.

For my parents, I love you very much and I am extremely lucky to have all three of you.

To my sister, Tracy, thank you will never be enough for your unconditional love and support, but that won't stop me from saying it every chance I get. Thank you.

My adoring husband John, there are not enough pages in this book to express my love and gratitude for your encouragement and your presence in my life. I will show you every day, just how grateful I am.

For my daughters, Alexa, Allison and Avery, speak up and be heard. I love you.

Table of Contents

We never talked about sex in my house. I don't really know why, we just didn't. I am the youngest of five children and was raised in a catholic home. My parents divorced when I was four, after nearly twenty years of marriage, and my mother remarried when I was seven. Despite the big "D", my three parents were very respectful of one another. No one ever spoke ill of another, and if there were bad feelings amongst them, I never knew about it.

My mother took us to church every Sunday. I don't know if this was a contributing factor to the lack of discussion of sex in my home, but I distinctly remember believing that I would go to Hell if I was curious about or explored my own body. Still, there was no sit down informative session about sex.

As we got older, Mom would send my sister and me to church on our own. We did attend a few times, in the beginning, but most times we just sat on the swings at the park. We talked about everything; those times with my sister are some of my fondest memories.

Now, the short version of the story is, I struggled with relationships for the very beginning. This certainly could have been due to raging hormones during the pubescent years, but it might have been the constant state of confusion I seem to remember always being in. I didn't have a lot of friends, and the friends I did have were manipulative and conditional. I didn't know how to deal with difficult relationships or how to end relationships without fear.

I don't know if I was any worse or better off than anyone else, I just have a better understanding of it today. My feelings were normal; I just wish I had known that at the time. I wish someone had talked to me about all those things that are difficult to talk about.

Human sexuality is how people experience the erotic and express themselves as sexual beings. Once I realized that I wasn't "crazy" or "dirty" and that I was "normal" to explore my own body, it allowed me to have a greater understanding of sex, sexuality, intimacy and love.

That understanding has afforded me to finally experience healthy relationships, with myself and with my partner.

Prologue

I had never been to any in-home party…ever. Not a candle party, not a jewelry party, anything, until my friend invited me to an Athena's party. I got the email invitation and I wondered, "Athena's? What's that?" My friend emailed me back two words that would change my life: adult novelties.

I gasped! I was so excited I immediately typed back "they have parties for that? I am SO there". Now I know how I am, and I know how my friend is, and I knew some of her friends, but I didn't know them *that* well. I wasn't really sure what was going to happen at this party.

So the calendar flips to November and Saturday the sixth – the day of the party. I was still a little uncertain as to what it was going to be like. The consultant (or Goddess, as they are called) arrives; She enters and mixes in with the rest of the crowd. She didn't look any different. She didn't sound any different. She didn't act any different when she started showing products. She started with bathing and massage items, which we all passed around. She just made everyone feel comfortable. We were all just sitting around the living room and it wasn't weird or awkward at all.

After the presentation, it was time for us to place our orders. She carried stock, so we walked outside to this van that had all these bins filled with the items she just showed us available to take home that evening! I spent $126 without even buying a vibrator. She looked up at me as she tallied my order and asked "No toys?"

"Well, I just started seeing this guy" I explained to her, (I literally had just met my husband days before) "and I'm really not sure if he's going to be into any of this". She didn't hesitate, looked me right in the eye and said, "well if he's not into it, then you know he's not the guy for you". That struck me, and it stayed with me, it was like she knew me. I said, "You know what, you don't know how right you are".

She proceeded to ask me if I would be interested in booking a party, and as much as I would've liked to, I really didn't think anybody would come. But when she asked me if I'd be interested in being a Goddess, I thought, "this could be fun". I was sitting in this van full of sex toys talking to this woman who goes to parties, talks about sex and makes money.

Sounds like my kind of party.

So I did it. I joined Athena's and became a "Goddess" because it seemed like a productive way for me to spend every other weekend while my daughter was with her father, and a fun hobby where I could make a little money.

At one of my very first parties, I met an incredible woman. She was stunningly beautiful, sophisticated, poised and looked much younger than her fifty-seven years. She told me how she was brought up in a very conservative family and that she remained a virgin until the night of her wedding.

She told me she accepted early on that sex was part of her marital duties in order to please her husband. She confessed that she never enjoyed it. She never experienced an orgasm. Later on in her marriage she accepted that her husband would keep a mistress and then, after nearly thirty years of marriage, he left her for a younger woman.

She said she spent years blaming herself. She wondered what was wrong with her, what did she do wrong, what could she have done differently. She fell into a deep depression and spent years in therapy.

She realized that there was nothing wrong with her. She was starting to experience life again and was so glad she came that night because she had never been to a sex toy party.

She wanted to purchase the most expensive toy I had, though she confessed she had never used a vibrator before. I was concerned that if she didn't love it, it may turn her away from toys all together. Instead I guided her to three different, middle of the road priced items, instead. Each was different and I told her this would give her more variety and she could experiment and get familiar with what she liked or didn't like. She thanked me with a hug, and left with her toys.

The next day I got a phone call:

"I think I had my very first orgasm!" I heard a bit of shock and excitement in the voice on the other end. "Thank you" she proclaimed in a deeply emotional tone. "Thank you so much" she continued "Thank you."

At that moment, I realized I was part of something much bigger than me. I did a lot more than just sell dildos. I entertained. I educated. I empowered.

I was a Goddess.

When I decided to write this book, I was concerned about some of the negative resistance I could encounter.

I had already started to plan the party for the book's release. I was looking forward to a big gala at a brand new, trendy place that had recently opened in my town. It had high ceilings, gorgeous outdoor fireplaces and valet parking. A few days after I had called to inquire about hosting my event, I received the following email:

Good afternoon Jenifer,

Thank you for your interest in <name of venue>. I have had a chance to run this by the Marketing Director etc. We will not be able to hold your party here at <name of venue> due to the nature of the content. Thank you for your time and effort, and I wish you luck in the future with your book launch!

I couldn't believe it. It really bothered me at first, but when I talked about it, I gained support from followers and realized that this denial was only reinforcement that this book needed to be written.

Once I finally secured a location, I contacted my local newspaper to run an ad promoting the event. Nothing fancy, just a photo of the book cover with the event details to support a local author. I spoke to a woman that said she loved the design, declaring it was beautiful and tasteful. She believed she would have no problem running my ad, but said she did need to get approval first. Then I get the email:

Good morning Jenifer:

Unfortunately, I have not been given permission to run an ad for you.

I apologize for any inconvenience and wish you the best of luck with your book.

I thought about the very content that is within these pages. The fear and shame that surrounds talking about sex, sexuality and masturbation. The more I met with opposition, the more I was reminded that I needed to continue and get it done.

Because I am a Goddess.

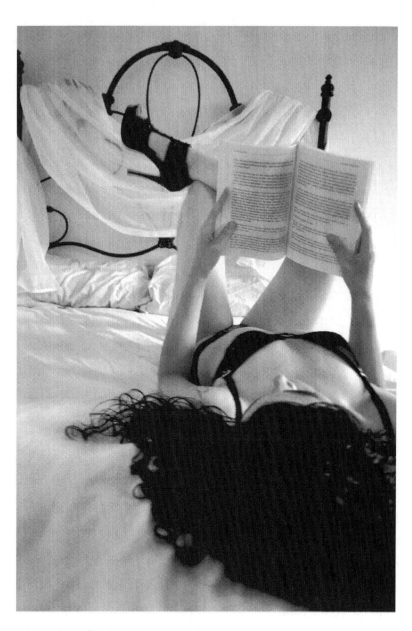

Photo by Elle Cei Photography

CHAPTER 1

Leave your baggage at the door
7 Questions to ask yourself

Ask yourself how you learned about sex:

1. How old were you when you first learned about sex?

2. Who was the first person to talk to you about sex?

3. Were you ever given any misinformation about sex?

4. Did anyone ever talk to you about masturbation?

5. How old were you when you first had sex?

6. Was your first sexual experience pleasurable?

7. Did anyone teach you about safe sex?

We are sexual beings. Our sexuality is present when we are born and it is with us until we die. It is an integral part our identity and humanity and affects who we are and how we express ourselves as sexual beings. Much of what you think you know about sex and sexuality may be inaccurate as well as confusing. A basic understanding of sex and sexuality can sort out myth from fact and help us all enjoy our lives more.

Many in our society still struggle with discussing the topic of sex with their kids, their parents, their friends, and even their partner. Sex is not a dirty word. If we don't speak of it, if we instead whisper it or spell it out, we are implying that there's something wrong with sex...both the word as well as the act. Sex and sexuality need to be discussed openly and honestly in order to remove the stigma and taboo that continues to hang over it in the 21st century.

When I first started conducting in-home parties in 2004, I spoke to so many women (and some men as well), that shared similar stories. Some were as young as eighteen and some were as experienced as sixty-four, but most said the same thing to varying degrees: Very few talked about sex in the home.

One of my very first customers was a young woman in her mid-twenties. She was a little uncomfortable passing sex toys around the room like they were hors d'oeuvres. I could understand that. She would hold it with two fingers as it came around to her and pass it off quickly the same way while her friends giggled. When it came time for her to order, I assured her the process was completely confidential, and that she could ask me anything about any of the items I showed.

She freely shared her story with me. She said that she first learned about sex at age nine. While in fifth grade, she was forced into total embarrassment along with the rest of the female students when they had to watch "The Video" about menstruation and puberty. Feeling a little confused and unsure after the viewing, she went to her older sister because she didn't feel comfortable talking to her mother.

I didn't ask her how much older her sister was, or why she wasn't comfortable talking to her Mother. She did mention that her sister probably didn't know much more than she did at the time. In fact, her lack of accurate information at that time probably contributed to her lack of curiosity about sex - until she was twelve.

With the onset of puberty and raging hormones one's body can seem like it's out of control and if you don't know what's happening, it is even harder to understand. This young lady was smart though. Still not comfortable talking to her mother, and not having a lot of faith in her sister's wisdom, she went off on her own...to the library. She wanted to be informed.

A repeat customer at another party in her mid-forties told me of her catholic upbringing. "My mother told me about my period, and don't have sex till you're married" she said. Even as she was about to marry, there was no real talk about sex, much less the orgasm.

She continued to share with me that she now has an empowered sex life with her second husband. She said that I was very easy to talk too. She felt comfortable with me and that I was approachable. I'm a Mom like her that just happens to have an interesting job.

One thirty-something customer told me how she found her Dad's Playboy Magazine when she was ten. She was very curious about how her body would soon develop, so she took it to the bathroom in order to have a little more privacy and to avoid being caught. She was very intrigued and enjoyed the articles as much as the photographs. However, this created a moral dilemma - stealing was a sin, and so was masturbation.

Almost the entire summer passed before her dad finally realized it was his little princess who had lifted his favorite publication. Having four brothers, she thought her dad would assume it was one of them who took it. When she was confronted, she caved and she told the truth and confessed to everything: Taking the magazine, reading the articles, liking the pictures, and looking at them while she touched herself because it made her feel good.

Unfortunately her father was not prepared to hear such honesty from his little girl. Maybe he should have called on mom for some backup, but instead her father just said, "OK, I won't tell your Mother about this".

Because of the way he handled it, she felt tremendous guilt and shame. "Was I not supposed to like it?" she wondered. Now she was confused and she couldn't even talk to her father or her mother about it.

A tall, confident and beautiful woman, twenty-nine, who had never been married once told me, "I was always told sex is to be with someone you love. Sex should be special. It's the most amazing experience two people can share".

Her confidence and poise faded as she continued to share her story. She conveyed her sadness over losing her virginity at a very young age; promiscuity and multiple partners before the age of twenty. She had very low self-esteem as a young girl and when a boy was nice to her, she perceived that as love, so she would have sex with him.

Sex is not love. That was the lesson that had to be re-programmed in her brain. As a young adult she emerged from her negative sexual experiences, though she admitted that she wished she had her first vibrator at fourteen and her first boyfriend at twenty-five.

One time, a lovely young lady aged twenty-two came in and said, "I'm boring". I assured her she was not, regardless of what she did or did not purchase. She insisted that she was, explaining that she didn't even like sex.

She had never had a pleasurable sexual experience. "Good girls don't" was the lesson taught in her home. She considered herself to be a "good" girl because she got good grades and stayed out of trouble. She gave in to her first boyfriend when she was just seventeen because she could no longer take the pressure to have sex from her peers. The experience was awkward, uncomfortable and painful. She did not communicate her discomfort because she was afraid she would hurt his feelings and he would break up with her.

One woman that stands out was the first one to tell me, "I have tons of these" referring to the many sex toys of her personal collection. She had a very open relationship with both of her parents who had informed her of the responsibilities that go along with sex, the emotional maturity, as well as the precautions to take in order to prevent pregnancy and to protect herself from sexually transmitted diseases (STDs). These may have been scare tactics, but she didn't mind. Though her parents didn't disclose the benefits of masturbation, she deemed it as the safest sex there is.

I was surprised initially that so many people would so readily open up to me and share these intimate details of their lives. Maybe they saw that I was well-trained and very professional, and therefore viewed me as a "Sexpert" (an expert on the subject of sex and sexuality), especially after giving my tasteful presentation and after sharing various sex statistics and facts. My job is to make everyone feel comfortable. Mission accomplished.

Take a minute to think about the seven questions at the start of this chapter. The age and manner that you first learn about sex is important. Parents have a hard time seeing their children as sexual beings. If you are a parent yourself, you may have a deeper appreciation for why that is.

Some people are comfortable and confident talking with their kids about sex and sexuality while others may find it difficult. If your parents told you a lot or a little, gave you accurate information or were just plain wrong at least give them an "A" for effort if they even made an attempt. Most people that I spoke to learned about sex from someone other than their parents; a sibling, a babysitter, a friend or someone the same age as they were who knew as little (or less) then they did. The misinformation shared was passed around like an STD.

Let's not dwell on the past and/or all of the misinformation received growing up. You are reading this book because you want to be more comfortable with your sexuality, so give yourself a pat on the back. "Leave your baggage at the door" and we'll start from scratch. By the end of this chapter, you may feel like you had a crash course in sex education. That's quite alright. In fact, that would be a good thing.

Sexuality includes many different things, the body being just the start. All of its parts and systems, together with sexual and reproductive anatomy are only the beginning. It's a good start (and good practice) to use the correct names for all body parts including sex and reproductive organs.

Several of us grow up with an inaccurate sexual vocabulary. Children are seldom taught the correct names for genitalia, and this can extend to sexual behaviors, orientations and identities as they get older. For instance, when you say "winky" it leaves the impression that the appropriate word (penis) is somehow not acceptable and possibly even offensive. And don't even get me started on Mommy's pet names for the Vagina!

While this seems to be changing with the volume of sexual content in the media and online, there are still people who have a hard time talking about sex because they just don't know the words they want to use in order to express what they want to say.

Having a basic sexual vocabulary will make it easier to talk about sex. It will also be reassuring to discover that there are words for how we feel and others that describe these feelings and experiences.

Think back to when you were a kid, when we had songs that taught us the names of certain body parts. "Head, shoulders, knees and toes (knees and toes)" was a popular preschool favorite. Sing along and point to the corresponding body parts. "Head, and shoulders, knees and…wait a minute, I think you skipped a few…

While I am not suggesting that we ban this song in our public schools, it does inadvertently suggest that those parts in between our shoulders and knees are not worth mentioning.

Perhaps in a private and safe environment those lyrics could be, "lips, breast, vagina, anus (vagina, anus) for the girls and "lips, penis, scrotum, anus (scrotum, anus) for the boys.

According to Planned Parenthood, children between the ages of three and five should know and understand biological sex, whether we are male, female or intersex. Again, if you think about a pre-school class, a teacher can ask the boys to sit in one circle and the girls to sit in another circle. The teacher may then show the class pictures of adults in order to understand the difference between genders and grown-up boys and grown-up girls, more commonly referred to as men and women.

Remember when you were a kid and it didn't matter if your playmates were boys or girls? You may be too young to remember that but kids will play with other kids regardless of sex. As they get older and when they start to go to school kids may then prefer to socialize with playmates of their own sex. Sometimes there are a few who prefer the opposite sex. This is totally OK and normal. As kids identify with gender, they'll develop feelings and become comfortable (or uncomfortable) with their gender. This is all part of the process in understanding gender identity.

Gender identity is the comfort with and the feelings about one's gender. An individual who may not be comfortable with their own gender may start to doubt their gender selection. AM I NORMAL? These emotional changes are common during puberty, when girls and boys mature physically and sexually — when a girl is becoming a woman and a boy is becoming a man.

Sometimes these are the early developments of sexual orientation, whether one is straight, lesbian, gay or bisexual.

Accept that human sexuality and your own sexual feelings are an important and natural part of your life. People have sex for pleasure, not only to make babies. Understanding sexuality also includes the biology of the fertility cycle, understanding how pregnancy happens, and how to prevent pregnancy by practicing safe sex.

Sexuality is a positive piece of one's personality. There are numerous different and normal ways to have sex play and express one's sexuality. People can form several kinds of sexual relationships, including opposite-sex and same-sex partnerships.

The way we feel about our sex, gender and orientation as a whole makes up our sexual identity. Sometimes those feelings about who we are sexually are not always be positive. This could be because we received some inaccurate, negative, or NO information about sexuality. If we nurture our children's sexual identity, and educate them to be comfortable about their bodies, maybe there would not be so much angst when people (at any age) question their own sexual identity.

It is still so hard for me to believe. Usually one or two at every party is extremely comfortable with opening up about her sexual issues and challenges. "I didn't know that" they whisper to me, the only other person in the room. Because nobody ever told them…seriously.

Values, attitudes, beliefs, and ideals about life, love and sexual relationships are all part of, and NORMAL, ways to express one's sexuality. Sexual activities and the ways in which we have sex, including masturbation and sexual intercourse, are ways to experience sexuality, which should also be considered normal.

I cannot even tell you how many times a woman at one of my parties told me their story about how their faith would make them feel guilt or shame (or both) about touching their own body. That is was a "SIN" to touch yourself. I remember one guest in particular who shared her fear growing up, "That's why he (God) made it feel so good, to tempt you, to see if you can resist".

Sexuality and the ways we experience and express it are influenced by biology. Our emotional lives, family lives, culture and our status in our culture, ethical, religious and spiritual upbringing and experiences all play a part in that influence as well. There is a great deal of contributing factors in how we learn to express ourselves sexually. If our ethical and spiritual upbringings clash with our biology and the status in our culture, this can create sexual conflict...and more worry, doubt, guilt or shame that there is something wrong with us...that we are not normal.

Love should make people feel good, safe and wanted. Your body belongs to you, and no one has the right to touch you without your permission. Open and honest communication and talking about sex and sexuality are fundamental to understanding healthy relationships. This will prove helpful on how to recognize and protect yourself against possible sexual abuse and its dangers.

Sexual predators may seem kind, giving, and loving. They may even be friends or family members.

Understanding sexuality is a lifelong process, especially if you had the misgivings, misunderstandings and disbeliefs about how you were supposed to feel about your body. Growing up you had to cover up immediately after getting out of the shower or tub. No one could walk around the house naked. As soon as we got clothes we would be covered up. Many people, children and adults, experience some sort of shame over their bodies. These adolescent experiences are normal, but no one is really telling these kids they are normal and reinforcing it. Those kids cannot get past feeling dirty or bad. Those kids grow up and it is hard to have healthy relationships as an adult, with another adult.

We can help our children gain this understanding by giving them age-appropriate information so that they can break the cycle, and become adults that can talk about sex, because sex is not a dirty word. Understanding our sexuality will help us enjoy our lives more, and who doesn't want that?

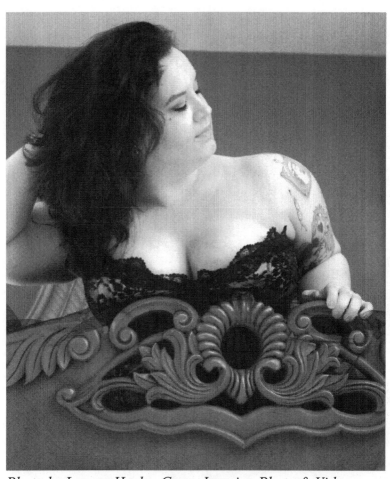

Photo by Lauren Healey Green Imaging Photo & Video

CHAPTER 2

Be sensual in your own skin

Whether you're a size 2 or 22

In order to be comfortable with your sexuality, you need to be comfortable with how you look. How do you feel when you look in the mirror? Do you stand up straight and smile, or do you start criticizing the things you wish you could change? What do you think other people think about how you look? Do others people's opinions matter to you?

Body image is more about how we see our own body than how someone else sees it. Depending on whether or not someone has a positive or a negative body image, it can affect one's comfort with their own sexuality.

Do you ever avoid activities like exercising, going to the beach or having sex because you are uncomfortable showing your body? How do you usually reply when people compliment how you look? Can you list your three favorite things about your body?

We all have feelings about the way we look, and we have ideas about what others think about our looks. Overall body image can range from very positive to very negative. You may feel good about certain parts of your body and not as good about others, and that's totally normal. Body image is also how you feel in your body, whether you feel strong, confident, able, good-looking, and in control or reserved, unattractive and insecure.

Men and women of all ages can struggle with body image. People do not develop their body image all on their own. Messages received from family, friends, church, society, and the media, etc. are all powerful influences that can mold how you see yourself sexually.

Positive and negative messages about our bodies from family and friends are conveyed all the time — starting at a very young age. For example, we may develop a love of exercise and a sense of being strong and capable if our parents share their own enjoyment of physical activity with us. On the other hand, we may develop a negative body image if our parents criticize the way we look.

According to The National Eating Disorders Association and Screening for Mental Health, the average U.S. woman is 5'4" and weighs 140 pounds whereas the average U.S. model is 5'11" and weighs 117 pounds. Two out of five women and one out of five men would trade three to five years of their life to achieve their weight goals.

Body image is not limited to how you think you look. How you *feel* and what you *think* when you look at yourself in the mirror, as well as how you presume other people see you, plays a pivotal role in understanding sexuality. Everyone's body is different. Each one is unique and they all come in different sizes, shapes and colors. Your Body belongs to you.

How you feel about your body and all of its moving parts contributes to your total body image. Your build and your legs, your nose and your ears, your stomach and your feet, the color of your skin and the texture of your hair all play a role in your body image. This includes your sex organs as well. The vagina and vulva, breasts, penis.

Appreciate that boys and men's bodies differ, just as girls and women's bodies differ. There is a natural curiosity about those differences amongst young children, thus the reason we need to communicate with them at the appropriate age.

One woman shared a story with me about when she was growing up. From the time she was about seven to well into her teenage years, she was taller than most of her classmates - a lot taller, and very thin. Although she was very beautiful, her father often referred to her as "stretch" or "the giant". She said she always felt awkward, not because of her height, but because of how her father always referred to her by her unique physique instead of her name.

An older gentleman told me he used to wear his hair long when he was younger. His mother constantly commented on his "long and greasy" hair to which he would always respond with a pleasant, "Mom, I just washed it". She often complained that he looked a hippie, a musician, a deadbeat or a druggie and that it made him unattractive.

While I'm certain parents never intend to plant these negative messages in their children's heads, these are the messages that leave an impression.

We also get ideas about body image from television, movies, magazines, the internet and other media outlets. Our society seems to be obsessed with the commercialized image of the ideal body. Many of the beliefs we have about the way people "should" look comes from the models and celebrities we see in the media.

But models and celebrities do not look like most people, and most of those images we see are edited, photo-shopped, blurred or otherwise manufactured to look the way they do.

Well, beauty truly is only skin deep, and perfection is in the eye of the beholder. The photographer, the make-up artist and the director only create what most people want to see. While no body is perfect, yours is yours and perfect for you. It is the media that exploits our insecurities. Individuals that are uncomfortable with their appearance are the ones buying these magazines with tips on how to have a better body/career/marriage/sex/life. Some just become depressed or develop self-esteem issues. These images of perfection are unrealistic and unattainable; the majority of fashion models have very different builds and are thinner than 98% of American women.

All we have to do is look around — the bodies in the real world are much more diverse and unique than those we see in the media.

We need to understand and recognize how body image is portrayed in the media — and how to control how much the media shapes what we think and how we feel about own body. This would build self-esteem and confidence about how we feel about ourselves as people and contributes to how we feel about our bodies, which would then lead to sexual empowerment.

Body image is also influenced by the natural aging process and our life experience. We have different feelings about our bodies when they change. Certain times in life, such as puberty or menopause and andropause, are key times when a person's body image may change. If people are hurt, sick, or disabled, their body images may be affected, too.

Our emotional state also influences our body image. When work or relationships become stressful, many people notice that their body image can be affected. Someone may lose their job or get passed over promotion and develop a negative body image while a raise or a new position may improve self-esteem and cultivate a positive body image.

People who accept the way they look and who feel good about their bodies most of the time have a positive body image. Their appearance may not match their family's ideals or the ideals in the media, but they have learned to be proud of the way they look.

You do not have to be thin or tall or have any other specific physical traits to have a positive body image. It does not matter what you look like from the outside. Having a positive body image is about being happy about the way YOU feel about the way YOU look.

Have you put on a new outfit and then stood there looking at yourself in the mirror? You stand up straight and turn to one side, then you turn to the other, and finally you turn your head over your shoulder to see how you look from behind. You run your hands down your waist over your hips once or twice, maybe past your stomach or over your butt because it flatters every curve of your body and you *feel* really good because you *look* really good?

Did you ever go to the hairdresser and have your hair colored a few shades darker or lighter? Or maybe you just a got a regular haircut or went with a bold new style. You turn your head to see it from all angles. You run your fingers through your hair because it feels so good. Then you walk out of the salon with your head held a little bit higher.

That same confidence and self-esteem can accompany a new perfume, cologne, or maybe even jewelry; or maybe it was from a day at the spa or something as simple as a good night's sleep. A compliment from a lover-or a stranger could even cause it. When you feel good, you are good. When you feel you look great, that in turn makes you feel great.

You may feel that same euphoria after mind blowing sex, too. Think about the morning after, Mom and Dad are smiling as everyone is trying to get out the door for work and school. Kinder words are spoken; Mom has more patience, a little bounce in her step.

Anyone can have mind blowing sex. You don't have to be a lingerie model to put on a sexy night gown and feel like one. When you *feel* sexy, you *are* sexy, no matter what size.

Part of having a positive body image is thinking about the way you physically feel and what your body can do — not just the way you look. For example, people who can easily climb stairs may have a better body image than people who struggle climbing them.

Having a positive body image also means that you see yourself as you really are. Many people with a positive body image know that certain parts of their body may not be the same as someone else's, but they accept, appreciate, and even love the differences.

Even the most confident and secure may see a few things they would change if given the opportunity, but continue to focus on what is beautiful and unique. Beauty is inside and out...so is confidence and sensuality. It's what makes us who we are and what makes us comfortable in our own skin.

People with a positive body image also understand that how they look does not determine their self-worth. They understand that to be truly comfortable in your own skin, you have to be comfortable with who you are. This includes comfort and confidence with who we are as somebody, not just some body.

Negative body image develops when someone feels his or her body does not measure up to family, social, or media ideals. Many people feel as if they don't measure up — especially when they measure themselves against the impossible standards of beauty commonly depicted in the media.

Of all the people I interviewed for this book, not ONE was proud of their physical appearance. Though most were OK with what they see in the mirror, not ONE considered their body to be beautiful. Try this experiment: Stand in front of a mirror (clothing is optional) and see how long before you start to notice things you don't like or wish you could change about your body.

Unlike people with a positive body image, people with a negative body image are often very dissatisfied with more than just their physical appearance. They may not even see themselves as they truly are, and have lower self-esteem and even be unhappy in other aspects of their life.

If you have a negative body image, you may feel self-conscious or awkward, and you may feel shame about your body. We may all feel this way about our bodies and ourselves from time to time — and that's normal. But if you have negative thoughts about the way you look or the way you think other people see you most of the time, you may have a problem, and it could be serious. Having a negative body image can have a harmful effect on one's health and well-being, and you may want to talk with a professional counselor.

Having a long-lasting negative body image can affect both your mental **and** physical health. People who have a long-lasting negative body image are more likely to have anxiety, depression, low self-esteem, shame, and trouble concentrating.

They are also more likely to take risks with their sexual health, cut themselves off from being with other people socially, and stop doing healthy activities that require them to show their bodies, (such as exercising, having sex, going to the doctor, or swimming).

Negative body image, depression and low self-esteem can cause one to suffer from serious mental health problems, such as anorexia, bulimia, over-exercising, or overeating. These disorders can be very serious.

There is a lot you can do to improve your body image, even without changing your body. Remember, body image is not about how you look, but how you feel about the way you look.

Some people choose to change the way they feel about their bodies. Many times, talking about the way you feel with someone that you trust (such as a friend or family member) can help. Professional help from a therapist may also be useful. Talking about your negative feelings and developing new ways to think about your body and your self-worth is a good way to address a negative body image.

Think differently about your body. Pay attention to the times when you feel bad about your body. Did you just weigh yourself? Did you just read a magazine? Did you just talk to a friend or family member who is negative about her or his image?

People may choose to change their appearance in many ways, and for a variety of reasons. If you want to change the way you look, be sure that you have realistic expectations. If you have a negative body image, it is important to deal with the mental and emotional aspects of it in order for any physical changes to be truly successful.

Some people choose to make lifestyle changes, such as adopting a specific diet and an exercise program in order to lose weight, gain muscle, or change their bodies in other ways. Often, this can be a healthy choice. If you are planning to make a considerable change in your lifestyle, it can be a good idea to talk to a health care provider who can advise you about the healthiest way to do so.

People also change their looks in other ways, such as coloring or processing their hair, or using products to change the appearance of their skin. Some changes can boost self-esteem and body image, and some changes may not be as effective. The key is to have realistic expectations about how much changing your appearance can change how you feel about yourself.

So maybe you could stand to lose a few pounds like most of the general population in America. Maybe you wish you were taller, had lighter hair, or more hair, a bigger penis or bigger boobs. Some things are within your control (such as your weight) and some are not (though height can be modified with heels). Be happy and accepting of your own body as well as yourself.

Some people do not accept their own bodies and instead choose to have plastic surgery to change what they don't like. This is one way to address a negative body image, but changing a body part does not necessarily change the way a person feels.

If you are planning to make a drastic change in the way you look, you may want to think about any possible health consequences. It can be a good idea to talk about your plans with a trusted friend, family member or health care provider.

Especially for Teens - The preteen and teenage years are a time when bodies change rapidly, and young people's body image also changes. This is also a time when many people — especially young women — struggle with a negative body image.

Body image is an important part of your sexual health. People who feel comfortable in their bodies are more likely than others to make healthy sexual decisions, like protecting their health by using condoms. Individuals who feel comfortable with their sex organs are more likely to be comfortable talking openly about sex with a partner. Others who feel ashamed of their bodies, including their sex organs, may not feel confident and strong enough to make healthy sexual decisions.

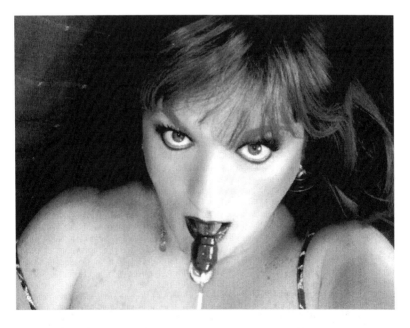

Photo by Alex Marin

CHAPTER 3

Let your fingers do the walking

Self-exploration

Masturbation refers to touching one's own body, including sex organs, for pleasure. Other terms used to describe masturbation include self-love, solo sex or self-pleasuring. It is a NORMAL process in which there is manual or mechanical stimulation of the sex organs for the purpose of sexual gratification. Masturbation often (but not always) leads to orgasm and can be accompanied by sexual fantasies.

Like sex, masturbation is also considered by some to be a bad word and a forbidden topic for discussion. Harmful myths about masturbation still exist that can cause some people to feel uncomfortable about it. These myths can create feelings of guilt, shame and fear...just like sex and sexuality can, which was discussed in chapter 1.

In the late 1940's and early 1950's Alfred Kinsey published The Kinsey Reports, which were the results of over 15 years of research in human sexual behavior. His studies revealed that approximately 95% of males and 60% of females had masturbated.

The National Health and Social Life Survey and other research conducted confirm between 48-95% of people masturbate.

The American medical community pronounced masturbation as normal in the 1972 publication Human Sexuality.

Not only is masturbation NORMAL, it is POSITIVE. Unfortunately, masturbation (like sex) and its benefits are rarely discussed as a healthy topic. So if no one is talking about it because the belief is that you shouldn't do it, the silence sends a negative message. Even if it is discussed, the message could still be a negative one; like it's forbidden or even harmful to touch your body.

In fact, the word origin and history, as defined by the Online Etymology Dictionary (© 2010 Douglas Harper), even state the words "defilement" and "dishonor"

masturbation 1766, *from Mod.L. masturbationem , from L. masturbatus , pp. of masturbari* . The long-standing speculation is that this is altered (probably by influence of turbare "to stir up") *from *manstuprare , from manu , abl. of manus* "hand" (see manual) + *stuprare* "defile" (oneself), *from stuprum* "defilement, dishonor," *related to stupere* "to be stunned, stupefied" (see stupid). But perhaps the first element represents an unattested **mazdo-* "penis." An earlier technical word for this was Onanism (q.v.).

Perhaps you once heard that masturbation is harmful or that it leads to strange behavior. Compounded with some of the many common myths about masturbation that (unfortunately) still exist today, it's no wonder that the topic generates such feelings and confusion. The myths, however, are simply not true.

Masturbation does NOT lead to blindness or cause hair to grow on the palm of your hands. It does NOT make sex organs shrink or grow, it does NOT stunt growth, either. Masturbation does NOT cause infertility or lead to mental illness. It does NOT cause injury or harm and it does NOT make you gay. Masturbation does NOT "ruin" a person for sex with a partner.

More adverse perceptions can be the result of personal experience. A young man once told me he was traumatized when his father returned home early from work and entered his bedroom while he was masturbating. His father was embarrassed and quickly exited his son's room, but after that he often teased him that he would "yank it right off" if he continued to do "that".

The fact is, self-exploration is a natural and common activity that plays a key part in becoming comfortable with your sexuality. Our bodies are amazing and complex and each one of them is beautiful and unique. It is natural to experiment with what feels good and we should be allowed to explore our own body freely without fear, anxiety, shame, embarrassment, remorse or guilt that it is wrong, socially unacceptable, or a mortal sin.

People may start masturbating at any time in their lives. Many children begin self-exploration as they grow and discover their changing bodies and often discover early on that it feels good to touch their genitals. Children usually begin masturbating long before puberty, though young children do not have sexual fantasies while masturbating. During adolescence is when it becomes more sexual.

Once again, it goes back to what we learn, and how we learn it, from an early age. We accept what we teach which is why it is important for children to learn that masturbation is normal and okay. They should also know to seek privacy when masturbating and that they should practice good hygiene, such as making sure their hands are clean beforehand. When children and young adults are taught that masturbation is normal, it creates a solid foundation for being comfortable with their sexuality and talking about sex as adults, and later as parents, thus breaking the cycle.

Some people think that others only masturbate when they do not have a sex partner. That is not true. Actually, people who have regular sex partners are more likely to masturbate than people without sex partners. With or without a partner, people masturbate for a variety of different reasons, such as to relieve sexual tension, achieve sexual pleasure, to experience sex when partners are unavailable, and to relax and fall asleep.

Many cultures and religions teach their young girls and women that sex is something you only do when you are married, or that it is something that is shared between one man and one woman, or that sex should be with someone you love, or for procreation and not recreation. The fact is, our bodies have a mind of their own. Our bodies can often show the physical signs of arousal and our minds have no say. If we are taught to resist or ignore these feelings, we are denying our own sexuality.

My friend told me a story of an older woman who, on the eve of her wedding, asked her mother what would happen on her wedding night, what could she expect. Her mother simply told her, "You'll find out".

Under the best circumstances, sex with a partner does take a certain amount of chemistry and coordination. So many women that shared their stories with me explained a first time experience that did not meet their expectations. This is not necessarily the fault of their partner; it was because they didn't know how to experience their own bodies.

Self-exploration is a common and safe kind of sex play that feels good...which is why it is often referred to as self-love. When you know how to experience your own body, what you like and what makes you feel good, it can be empowering. When you are in control of your own body as well as your emotions, then you can experience that with a partner.

Because sex is not love.

When the physical and emotional lines are blurred, that's when relationships can turn unhealthy. When women (and sometimes men as well) misinterpret or confuse the physical euphoria that can accompany sex play, the emotional cost can be high. Often times the relationships become co-dependent, with one partner thinking that this person must love them because they had sex with them.

When that earth-shattering, toe-curling, mind-blowing orgasm is first brought on by a partner, the lines can become blurred. Our minds may believe that only this person can make us feel this way. This can lead to unhealthy relationships for both men and women, particularly if someone has waited a long time to have sex with a partner and has not yet experienced self-pleasure.

Our bodies can have physical responses that our minds may not be able to control. Though the response may be somewhat primal, we are not animals and a certain amount of self-control needs to be exercised. The same can happen in reverse. Mentally, you may want to have to sex, but your body does not physically respond.

Getting to know your own body first, and learning about what feels good to you, can increase your chance of feeling sexual pleasure with sex partners. When you know what you like when it comes to sex, your comfort with sex increases. And when your confidence and comfort levels are high, it is easier to let your partner know what you like when it comes time to share it with someone else.

Touch is what causes our bodies to produce a hormone called oxytocin. Oxytocin promotes a desire to touch and be touched. It's an exciting merry-go-round that can have wonderful results. Oxytocin makes us feel good about the person who causes it to be released, and it causes a bonding between the two persons. Nursing a baby also produces oxytocin in both mother and child, and thus is a major part of what initially bonds a mother and her baby. Even thinking of someone we love can stimulate this hormone.

There are no health risks with self-pleasure, making it the safest sex there is. Skin irritation is possible, so always use plenty of lubrication to prevent that from happening. Everything is better when it's wetter (with or without a partner). Never, under any circumstances, use anything from your kitchen as lube, no cooking oil, no butter. No baby oil either, especially if you have a vagina, because these items were not designed for your vagina and will cause a yeast infection. No one has time for a yeast infection.

Men can use either a water-based or silicone-based lubricant. Women should use a water-based lube vaginally. Silicone is synthetic and while you can use it vaginally, your body can not naturally break it down, or flush out silicone. There is a great new water and silicone hybrid lubricant called Wet Synergy™ from Wet®, maker of the best-selling personal lubricants and intimacy products.

Do not insert anything inside your body that was not designed for that purpose....EVER! Again, anything from your kitchen or bathroom, or any household items or appliances that were not designed to go into the vagina or the anus should never enter your body. THAT'S WHAT SEX TOYS ARE FOR! That is what they were designed specifically for and, just like us, they come in all different shapes, sizes and colors.

As with any item you purchase, make sure to read all the directions that accompany your sex toys. All insertable toys should be used with lube. Clean your toys after each use. Make sure you know what your toy is made of and how to clean it. You can use antibacterial soap, but there is a toy cleaner product called "Mighty Tidy" that is an anti-bacterial, anti-microbial and anti-fungal spray that is designed specifically to clean sex toys. Never put your sex toys in the dishwasher (even if they are water-proof) and always take the batteries out of your motorized toys after use.

I have been selling relationship enhancement products since 2004, but I do so much more than sell sex toys. I noticed very quickly that people felt comfortable with me. I would always say, "If you have any questions, feel free to ask, if it's something that you prefer to ask me in private, ask me when you come into the ordering room". People would tell me if they never had a sex toy before, if they had them all, as well as ask what I could recommend for getting their sex drive back after having a baby, or how to introduce sex-toys to their partner.

Some would even tell me, "We don't need any of that stuff ". Well, it is never about "need"; it should be more about "want". There are times when sex can seem boring, mundane or routine, especially in long-term, monogamous relationships, and sometimes trying something new can spice up a relationship.

One of the myths about sex toys, similar to that of masturbation, is that a woman can become desensitized from using sex toys which is completely false. Actually, it is quite the opposite. Women who use sex toys understand their bodies on a deeper level. They become acutely aware of their pleasure center and the clitoris becomes more sensitive and responsive.

Jennifer Jolicoeur, the President of Athena's Home Novelties, shared a quote one time that, "Even the best carpenter uses power tools to get the job done!"

While some men may feel that their female partner will no longer want him or gain pleasure from his touch without sex toys, those men may need to be reassured that women sometimes use sex toys to spice things up...and at other times women don't use sex toys to spice it up!

Sex with yourself allows you to explore your body and the types of touch you like or don't like. It can help us learn how to get excited and how to achieve orgasm, so when it comes time to have sex with a partner, you can hit all of the right pleasure spots. Knowing how to experience self-pleasure and what feels good is another component of understanding sexuality.

Just like everything else in life that makes you feel good (what makes you feel good?), you do those things because you want to and because they make you feel good and it is important to feel good.

Unfortunately, many people experience shame or guilt about masturbating. When we don't talk about it, we give off the impression that it's not okay. That is the negative message that silence sends. When experienced at a young age, those feelings of shame transcend into adulthood. According to Planned Parenthood's website, approximately 50 percent of women and 50 percent of men who masturbate feel guilty about it.

Negative feelings about self-love, or any behavior for that matter, can threaten a person's physical health and well-being. Only you can decide what is healthy and right for you. If you feel ashamed or guilty about masturbating, then talking with a trusted friend, sexuality educator, counselor and/or therapist may help. It is NORMAL and talking about it is okay.

If you are concerned that you masturbate a lot, too much or too often, answer this question: Does masturbation interfere with your daily functioning, your job, your family, or your friends? If it does, then you may want to talk with a therapist about it.

You should not wait until your health and well-being are at risk to talk about sex. Don't let it get to that point. Sex is NOT a dirty word. Talk about it, embrace it, and practice it.

The skin is the largest organ on the human body, but it is the brain that is the largest sex organ. Experimentation with self-pleasure can be with the fingers, hands, or toys, and can be through internal or external stimulation. It is our brain that sends the signal that something feels good to the genitals and that is what triggers the blood flow.

Different people enjoy different things when they masturbate. Some people may engage in a "quickie" just to relieve sexual tension, while others may make a date for themselves, creating the space for it, and planning out where to do it.

Mutual Masturbation offers sexual pleasure and intimacy to partners that may not be quite ready for sexual intercourse. It allows people to experiment with what kind of touch they like, and to observe what kind of touch their partners like. It is also a great way to encourage communication and to practice verbalizing what you want, and what you like and don't like, in an intimate setting.

Women may stimulate all parts of their vulva, or just some, including the clitoris, the clitoral hood, the inner and outer labia, which all have erectile tissue. They may also stimulate the vaginal opening or canal, and/or the perineum or anus. Some women prefer rubbing near, but not on the clitoris because direct stimulation can be very intense. Men may stimulate the penis, scrotum, perineum and/or anus.

Men and women may also touch other sensitive areas of their bodies. There are nerve endings that can create erogenous zones (areas of the body that have heightened sensitivity), and people may experience pleasure by touching places like the breasts, nipples, thighs, the ear lobes or the lips.

Sex fantasies are normal and healthy. Fantasies may add to sexual excitement, alone or with a partner. Women and men may fantasize with their own thoughts or with erotic images or language — such as reading erotica or watching porn.

Not to mention the numerous health benefits of masturbation, like increasing self-esteem and improving body image. Masturbation also creates a sense of well-being and increases the ability to have orgasms. It helps with insomnia, improves sleep, releases sexual tension and reduces stress.

Masturbation provides a healthy sexual outlet for people who choose to abstain from sex play with another person, with no risk of disease or pregnancy.

It can also alleviate premenstrual tension, strengthen muscle tone in the pelvic and anal areas, reducing women's chances of involuntary urine leakage and uterine prolapse.

A number of studies have proven the benefits of self-pleasuring to mental, social and physical health and the health of our sexual relationships. People who feel good about their bodies, sex, and masturbation are more likely to protect themselves from sexually transmitted diseases and unintended pregnancy.

GOOD READING:

Tickle your fancy by Sadie Allison
Sex for one; the joy of self-love by Bettie Dodson
For Yourself: The Fullfillment of Female Sexuality by Lonnie Barbach
The Big Book of Masturbation by Martha Cornog

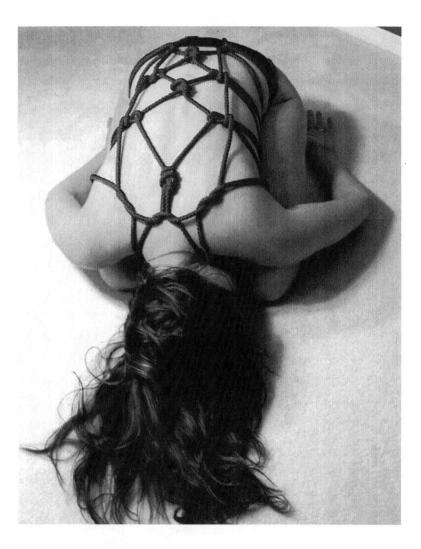

Photo by Christine Laplante

CHAPTER 4

They call it foreplay for a reason

It's supposed to be fun

The time will come when you will welcome a partner. While some people engage in open sexual relationships with more than one partner, I'd like to focus on getting comfortable with your own sexuality as well as a partner, so we will focus on a single partner for now.

I hope by now that you have a greater understanding of sexuality and sexual activity. Remember this includes a wide range of behaviors, and some sexual activities are more common than others. Talking with a partner about sexual behaviors (which we will explore more in chapter 5) may seem difficult, but it will help increase closeness, trust, and pleasure.

Sexual activity is an important way to connect with ourselves and with other people. Sexual activity is how we got here. It is normal and common and images of sex are all around us. It is also normal and common to have questions about sex and sexual activity, and it is okay to ask questions and to seek answers to those questions. While some people may shame you for asking, others will embrace you and they will provide comfort with the answers.

Foreplay is the physical and sexual stimulation (the touching, kissing, rubbing, and stroking), that often occurs in the excitement stage of sexual response.

Foreplay is not only FUN, but it should be a fundamental part of any sexual experience. Most men and women experienced in sex would agree that the best sexual encounters include long and sensuous foreplay. Getting there is half the fun, so do yourself and your partner a favor and don't take any shortcuts. A more attentive form of foreplay will bring increased pleasure to both partners, and make any sexual experience more satisfying.

Both partners need a little extra spice to get fully aroused and to achieve maximum pleasure. A man may need to prolong foreplay to become fully erect, and most women require ample foreplay in order to produce enough natural lubrication. Unless you are going for the standard 'quickie', there is no such thing as spending too much time on foreplay. The idea is not to move on to intercourse until both partners are fully aroused and just can't control their desires any longer.

Foreplay includes a wide range of activities such as massage, kissing and touching, caressing, stroking and oral sex (stimulating a partner's sex organs with the mouth) but the list is really only limited to your imagination. Foreplay is extremely important to good sex because it helps both partners enjoy sexual intercourse more and can help women achieve orgasm more often. Most woman need prolonged stimulation in order to reach complete arousal, and foreplay provides them with the required stimulus.

Foreplay is extremely important to a healthy relationship. When you let go of the woes of the day, the demands of the job, and the needs of the family, it paves the way to relaxation. Relaxation is essential to having a happy and healthy sex life because, often times, people do not achieve orgasm because of stress. Whether the foreplay is wild or mild, make the time and take the time to focus completely on your partner and allow them to focus completely on you.

There are no set rules or secret codes when it comes to foreplay. While it may seem similar to cracking a safe, the same combination may not get you in (pun intended) every time. It is not about running down a check list of kiss, touch, rub, lick, repeat in that order. It is about understanding what makes your partner feel good in order to make the experience pleasurable. There are many ways to please your partner and it all originates in the brain, before you hit the sheets.

A kind word goes a long way. Compliment your partner when they look nice. You can initiate foreplay and sex just by being genuine and telling your female partner, "You look beautiful" or even, "You are beautiful". Take a moment, look into your partner's eyes, and tell them something that you love you about them. Tell them what you want to do to them, - or better still, what you are going to do to them.

Sex talk or "talking dirty", while I don't like the term (because Sex is NOT a dirty word), is another form of foreplay that, thanks to 21st century technology, can occur anytime, even if you are not with your partner. There is phone sex and all kinds of cyber-sex. Email, instant messaging and online chat rooms have not only changed the way we meet our mates, (According to eHarmony.com, 1 in 4 relationships start from an on-line service) but how we initiate sex. Often times people do not verbalize their wants or desires out of fear or embarrassment, but sending an email is so easy.

Also easy is "Sexting", the act of sending sexually suggestive or explicit messages and/or photographs, primarily between mobile phones. The term was first popularized around 2005, and is a blend of the words *sex* and *texting*, where the latter is meant in the wide sense of sending a text, possibly with images. It can be very exciting to send a sexy text message to your partner to brighten up their work day. Or to receive one from your partner while you are out of town, perhaps with a photo of them alone in your bed with the simple caption "Waiting for you..."

Show your partner that you care about them and what they enjoy. If that means drawing them a bath after a long day, then do it. If it means sitting through that movie or TV show they really want to see, then do it. Make the most of it by sharing it with them, because the gesture can be quite the turn on, especially if you whisper in their ear, cuddle up to their body or draw hearts on the inside of their hand at the same time.

Arousal occurs with all five methods of perception (senses) hearing, sight, touch, smell and taste. Aside from the obvious, touching, there are the images we can create in our minds while reading. Erotica is considered sexually arousing imagery that is not considered pornographic, obscene, or offensive to the average person, such as Athena's compilation of erotic fantasies titled, "Goddess Bedtime Stories – 21 Tales to Keep You Up All Night".

Having your partner read to you allows you to hear their voice narrate the sexy scene you are imagining in your head. Looking at erotic images with your partner, or even taking photos of each other, is visually stimulating arousal, as is watching porn.

Foreplay doesn't have to start in the bedroom, either. The "romantic dinner" is often a prelude to sex, thus the 2 hour wait at any restaurant on Valentine's Day. While a romantic dinner out may be a treat, preparing a meal for your partner, especially if it's something they favor, is a kind gesture and a good way to set yourself up for *dessert.*

History is ripe with the pursuit of aphrodisiacs in many forms, particularly in food. Oysters are probably the food most associated with being an aphrodisiac, and most people are aware of their reputation for increasing sexual desire because of their high zinc content, which helps produce sperm and increases libido.

Honey, Sweet and sticky, is a great source of boron, a trace mineral that helps the body use and metabolize estrogen, the female sex hormone.

Studies have shown that this mineral may also enhance testosterone levels in the blood, the hormone responsible for promoting sex drive and orgasm in both men and women.

Pure chocolate, the king of natural aphrodisiacs, contains a host of compounds, including anandamide, the psyochoactive feel-good chemical, and PEA (phenylethylamine), the "love chemical," which releases dopamine in the pleasure centers of the brain and peaks during orgasm. PEA is said to help induce feelings of excitement, attraction and euphoria.

There are several erotic cookbooks available today. My favorites include "The New InterCourse" by Martha Hopkins, Randall Lockridge (Terrace Publishing), "50 Ways to Feed Your Lover" by Janeen A. Sarlin & Jennifer Rosenfeld Saltiel (William Morrow and Co.) and "Love on the Menu" by Linda Arsenault (Wine Appreciation Guild).

Some aromas can cause a greater effect on the body than the actual ingestion of food and can also be used as an aphrodisiac. It is said that aromas can help stimulate sexual arousal in both men and women. You should do your own research to see how aromatherapy can stimulate your sex life.

Studies have revealed that men show sexual desire from pumpkin and lavender odors, while almonds are said to induce passion in a woman. Women aroma studies have shown that the most popular arousal odor is with cucumbers and black licorice. Studies show that cherry odors showed a 13% increase in blood flow in women.

Surprisingly male colognes only had a 1% effect on vaginal blood flow. The smell of charcoal barbecue smoke lowers women's sexual drive by 18%. Some couples find that the natural smells of their partner are real turn-ons, and sometimes the partner is unhappy when the smells are washed away or covered up.

And then there are pheromones. Pheromones are a chemical substance secreted or excreted through the sweat glands that serve to influence the physiology or behavior of other members of the same species *(dictionary.com)*. These glands are located all over the body, but tend to be concentrated in underarms, the nipples (for both sexes), and the pubic region. In animals, sex pheromones indicate the availability of the female for breeding. While women who are on oral contraceptives, like birth control pills or other methods that suppress ovulation, may not omit the same sex scent, it is still very primal. That underlying scent in the air is what makes us perk up and alert.

Creating the right atmosphere for sexual intercourse is all about paying attention to detail. This is especially important at mature stages in a relationship. It's the little things, like making sure the room is warm, the lighting subdued, and that the appropriate soundtrack is playing. Once the mood is right, take the time to undress (yourself or your partner) slowly, because the removal of clothing can be a very exciting component of successful foreplay. Many find that undressing surges eroticism.

Foreplay should go slow; the kiss is usually the first physical expression of love and desire, but it is often forgotten during sexual intercourse. Kissing on the mouth, with the tongue and on body parts is a very sensual sex act. Touching, caressing, or even massaging your partner is always a nice way to get things started. Touching someone's body can be very erotic, even if it doesn't always start out that way.

Rubbing bodies together with or without clothing, oral sex and using sex toys together are all good forms of foreplay. Sex toys include, but are in no way limited to, items that require batteries.

Items such as a blindfold and a feather can enhance, or even change up, your foreplay. When you take away your partner's sense of sight, the other four senses become heightened in order to compensate. Tickling them lightly with a feather will become more erotic and exciting.

Other items like ropes or scarves can be sensual additions to your foreplay. While there are many beginner and advanced stages of rope work, a simple tie can be very new and exciting. Safety first: anytime you are experimenting with rope or other restraints, be certain to have scissors nearby, just in case. A rope corset can also be very sexy, to create as well as to see on your partner. Because rope serves as a conductor, you can also take your favorite massager or vibrator, touch the rope, and it will vibrate all along the rope.

Sex toys should not "ruin" the mood. They can improve a women's ability to achieve orgasm, and a man's ability to prolong, and the excitement they can add to foreplay is unlimited if you have an open mind. Again, this is where communication is crucial. Talk to your partner about the kinds of toys you want to use together and what you want to experiment with.

Don't limit your kissing to just foreplay, either. Continue during intercourse to kiss the different parts of your partner's body, not only their lips. Many women complain that their partner doesn't kiss long enough and rushes the movement directly to the genital area. Don't be shy to experiment on every part of the body, such as the neck and shoulders. Foreplay should be prolonged with more kissing and caressing. look your partner in the eyes.

Another reason foreplay is important is for the learning experience. Foreplay is the perfect time to discover what your partner likes because without that, you will never know what they really need to be fully stimulated. Don't be shy; ask for feedback or direction and also give your own. Both partners gain from good communication during foreplay and sex play. And if words fail you, SHOW or GUIDE your partner with what you like, and encourage them to do the same. Communication is absolutely necessary.

Foreplay is all too often, and sadly, neglected. Many women and men say they are just too busy, or too tired. They are constantly on the go, overbooking and spreading themselves too thin, dedicating more time to a job outside the home, the needs of the family and/or household, or the community. At the end of the day, many are just too exhausted to have sex and if they are not, the foreplay is often passed over.

That's why foreplay activities like massage and relaxation are pivotal to more enjoyable sex. One key reason people do not achieve orgasm is because of stress. Think about it: How many times are you just lying there...staring at the ceiling wondering if your partner is done yet?

Take your time. Relax; massage your partner's neck and shoulders if they have had a long day; perhaps their feet if they stand all day, or their hands. Make the time to connect (or re-connect) with them.

There are three, four or five steps in the sexual response cycle, (the pattern of the way we react to sexual stimulation) depending on who you talk to. Some or all of the steps are reached each time we have a sexual experience – with or without a partner. But we can stop at any step; we do not need to complete the cycle to be sexually fulfilled.

Sexual desire is sometimes referred to as libido. This inner sexual feeling does not require erotic stimulation and is the basic sensation that may initiate sexual activity and upon which sexual stimulation then builds. When sexual desire is low or absent, sexual functioning may be inadequate, unsatisfying, or absent.

Sexual excitement can last for a few minutes, extend for several hours, or even days. Excitement can consist of an increased level of muscle tension, an increased heart rate, flushed skin, hardened or erect nipples, and the onset of vasocongestion, which is the swelling of the clitoris and labia minora in women and the erection of the penis in men.

Other physical changes also occur. In the woman, the vaginal walls begin to produce a lubricating liquid, her uterus elevates and grows in size, and the breasts become larger. At the same time, the vagina swells and the muscle that surrounds the vaginal opening, called the pubococygeal muscle, or PC muscle, grows tighter.

Additional changes in men include elevation and swelling of the testicles, tightening of the scrotal sac, and secretion of a lubricating liquid by the Cowper's glands.

The plateau phase is characterized primarily by the intensification of all of the changes that occur during the excitement phase. During this period, the woman's clitoris may become so sensitive that it is painful to the touch. The plateau phase extends to the brink of orgasm, which initiates the reversal of all of the changes begun during the excitement phase. Some consider this to be an extension of the excitement phase.

The peak of sexual excitement, The Orgasm, is reached during the following phase.

We may not be aware of every change that happens in our bodies during sexual response. We experience each of these changes to varying degrees, depending on the unique nature of our bodies, and how much our bodies respond varies with our health and age and from one sexual experience to another. For example, women may have less lubrication as they get older or if they are taking certain medications.

Medications that can affect both arousal and orgasm in both men and women include many SSRIs (selective serotonin reuptake inhibitors) like Prozac, Paxil and Zoloft. Mood stabilizers like Clomipramine, Elavil, Marplan, Nardil, Parnate, Ativan and Thorazine, as well as some birth control pills. Tranquilizers like trazadone, valium, Xanax and Antihypertensives/medications for high blood pressure can also affect libido.

Some people believe that there are no bad lovers, and while no one is a champion right out of the gate when it comes to foreplay, communication and reassurance allow us to become better lovers. If you care about your partner, encourage them and be patient. If they care about you, they should make the effort.

If your partner shows little to no interest in wanting to take the time to please you, and sex is important to you, you may need to take a good look at the health of your relationship. I'll share this comment from a blog post:

"Anyone who does not believe in foreplay does not believe in fair play...and if they do not believe in foreplay OR fair play...back up and say "NO WAY!"

Foreplay is important for any sexual activity, including masturbation. Think about the Super Bowl, Opening Day or the Daytona 500. There is an elaborate display, visuals commemorating the event, a flashy musical performance on the infield, and sophisticated showcase to get you ready for the main event. There are driver introductions, the singing of our national anthem, a US military flyover, and then the most famous words in motorsports...

"Gentlemen, start your engines..."

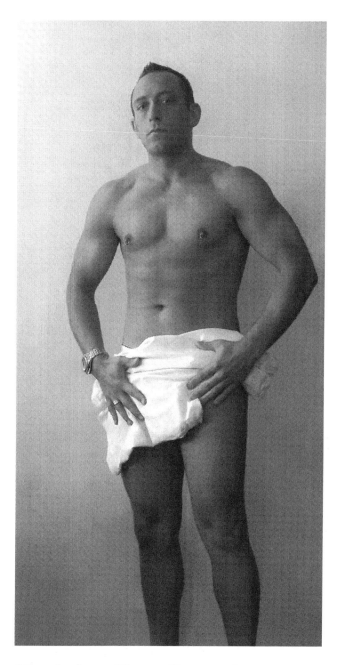

Photo by James Thomas Photography

CHAPTER 5

Speak up

Communication is key

Talking about sex is hard (sorry for the pun).

Most people have a difficult time talking about sex. It may have originated with the anxiety of asking their own parents about sex and may have evolved into the anxiety they may feel when their child asks them about sex. Some people may experience difficulty talking with their partner about a sexual issue, or asking a doctor a medical sex question.

Sex talk can feel anywhere from awkward to impossible. Understand that everyone has the right to feel embarrassed and/or uncomfortable and that is okay. Acknowledge that these are legitimate feelings and that you have the right to feel whatever it is that you feel and that it's perfectly normal.

What is NOT okay is to succumb to those fears and avoid talking about sex all together. We talk about everything else; leaving sex out is what gives the impression that it a forbidden subject. Silence about sex keeps us ignorant and potentially leads to negative sexual health outcomes, which could be anything from just having bad sex, unplanned pregnancy, acquiring sexually transmitted infections to abusive relationships and self-esteem issues. The lack of communication about sex also allows all of us to preserve sex myths that are rarely true but sound accurate in the absence of honest and open sexual communication.

Remember earlier when we talked about how people first learn about sex and who was the first person to have a conversation with them. Perhaps you're still waiting.

Parents have a tremendous and incredible responsibly. Parents nurture and protect their babies. They teach them how to walk and talk and how to eat healthy foods in order to grow up big and strong. Parents instruct their children on how to prevent cavities by brushing their teeth every day, and by seeing a dentist regularly. They educate them on how to be safe by looking both ways before crossing the street, and to protect themselves by wearing a helmet while riding a bike.

Some parents are concerned that if they talk to their children about sex, it may be perceived as giving some sort of permission or approval. It is important that parents communicate the facts as well as their own beliefs with what they hope for the children. Most teens say that their parents have the greatest influence on their sexual decision making.

Think about when you turned sixteen and you were finally old enough to drive. Did your Mom or Dad just hand you the keys? Of course not, you had to take a written test to get a learner's permit.

Someone probably popped the hood and showed you how to check the oil and where to add it if it was a few quarts low. Perhaps someone showed you how to check your fluids, you know, coolant, brake fluid, power steering fluid. Maybe Mom showed you where to fill it with gas and told you not to leave the gas cap on the top of the car. Dad may have been the one to show you where the spare is, and how to change a tire if you even get a flat.

And that's all before you even get in the driver's seat! Then what is the first lesson when you do get in the driver's seat? Buckle up and check your mirrors for safety. Then you may get the gas is on the right, brake is in the middle, clutch is on the left lesson.

Maybe you didn't get any of those lessons. Maybe you were told, "you can't learn how to drive until you get your license" to which you may have responded "I can't get a license till I learn how to drive".

Parents are the primary sexuality educators of their children. Parents want to help their children make healthier, safer, and better-informed decisions related to sex and sexuality, and teens really care about what their parents think, even if they don't always act like it.

Positive, open, honest and loving communication about sexuality help kids make better decisions and feel comfortable coming to their parents with questions and concerns. Most teens say it would be easier to postpone sexual activity if they were able to talk more openly about sex with their parents, and fewer still say that they have never had a conversation with their parents about the topic.

We are taught how to perform basic human behaviors, yet we're just supposed to know how to have sex. That is another common myth.

Some people believe that if they talk about sex, they will be judged or assumptions will be made about them. They think that if they ask questions they are speaking from experience, rather than looking for answers.

The lies we're told about sex present a huge barrier to good sexual communication. Many sex myths suggest that in order to be great lovers we need to be mind readers, not communicators. Communication isn't always verbal, but many experts believe that one of the secrets to great sex is an ability to talk about it. It is easier to learn how to be a good communicator and talk about sex than it is to learn to read minds.

The lies we are told or otherwise hear are as bad as silence when it comes to sex and they present a huge obstacle to healthy sexual communication.

Some may say that sex is natural and simple and that you should just know how to do it. While it is natural, yes, because we have to have sex in order to procreate and survive as a species; it is definitely not simple. Intercourse may be instinctual for some of us, but human sexuality is a whole lot more than just intercourse, and none of it really comes easy.

A number of people think that sex should be spontaneous and that you shouldn't talk about it, you should just do it. Sex is meant to be something fun and exciting that makes you feel good about your body and yourself. It is something that makes you feel loved and attended to. Why would planning it ever be a bad thing? Just like you plan a vacation or you discuss an upcoming date, wouldn't it be nice to know you're going to have sex at the end of the day?

Especially a particularly challenging day? Still the media, movies, and novels create the perception that the most exciting sex is the sex that "just happens" when you least expect it.

Here in the real world, sex rarely "just happens". While it is true that many couples do not discuss sex beforehand, that doesn't mean that one (or more likely both) partner isn't thinking about it, wondering when they're going to have it next, and fantasizing about what kind of sex it will be.

Our various fears about sex, such as rejection or disclosing socially "inappropriate" sexual desires or behavior, present substantial obstacles to good communication about sex. Most fears are often justified, since we live in a society of quick and cruel judgment of those who don't preserve the status quo. This is one more thing that makes it very difficult for us to talk about sex honestly with the people around us.

Several people have been raised with some of the negative sex beliefs discussed in chapter one, which can also prohibit us from talking about sex. The stigma surrounding the word itself is enough. When you get two people who each have their own negative sex beliefs the potential for miscommunication is multiplied.

Some negative sex beliefs can be very personal, like being told your body is ugly, dirty or should only be used for procreation, or even more general, like people who have sex end up single, depressed, or with a disease, etc. These beliefs act as strong deterrents to discussing sex.

We all have sexual feelings, though we may not always engage in sexual activity when we experience those feelings. When you have sex is a personal choice. Figuring out when you're ready for sex continues through life. People need to make decisions about sex in their teens, 20s, 30s, 40s, 50s, and beyond — every time a sexual situation develops.

A good sex life is one that keeps in balance with everything you're about — your health, education, career goals, relationships with other people, and your feelings about yourself.

When you're considering having sex, it is also important to consider how clear you can be with your partner about what you do and don't want to happen. Consider also that having sex may or may not change how you feel about yourself, both physically and emotionally.

It's also important to ask yourself if you are considering having sex because you want to or because someone is pressuring you? Will sex change your relationship with your partner?

Sometimes it's helpful to talk these kinds of decisions through with someone you trust — a parent, a friend, a professional counselor, or someone else who cares about you and what will be good for you. Ultimately, you want to be comfortable talking about sex with your sex partner, but if you can't, you should take a step back and explore why that is and if they are the person you want to have to have sex with.

Talking about sex with a partner or showing them what feels good and what excites us is an important part of a healthy and fulfilling sex life. Some people are able to share sexual desires and fantasies with a partner without embarrassment. For others, it may take some practice or be very challenging.

Communication is KEY - Talk about sex with your partner! Talk about the first time, the last time and the next time. Talk about being more spontaneous or adventurous or what you want. Many sex myths imply that to be a great lover, we need to be a great mind reader. The truth is a great lover is also a great communicator. Communication isn't always about talking, but one of the keys to great sex is the ability to discuss it.

I have helped thousands gain knowledge on how to talk about sex. I have taught none how to read minds.

To talk about sex, it helps to have some basic sex information. Unfortunately a lack of comprehensive sex education presents another hurdle to good sexual communication between partners. It's hard to know where to start a conversation about sex when you have no context within which to begin. Lacking basic information also makes talking about sex all the more scary, which leads to the fear and negative beliefs about sex we have mentioned.

Because so many of us have been told that sex is private, it may be more comfortable to have privacy to talk about sex. But many of us lack privacy, and our sexual communication suffers for it. Whether you have parents, kids or roommates, a door with no lock, thin walls, or worry about outsiders overhearing your conversation, makes having the conversation that much more challenging. Most people adapt and learn to make the best of the privacy they can find. If you carve out privacy both in terms of space and time; it will make your sexual communication go a little bit smoother.

Many people feel that the most uncomfortable and challenging conversations are the ones surrounding sexually transmitted infections, safer sex, and condoms.

Make sure to discuss safer sex with your partner before sex play starts. Talk about birth control if pregnancy is possible. People are much more likely to take risks when they don't plan ahead.

Any sex play that allows semen to enter the vagina could result in pregnancy. If you do not want to get pregnant or cause a pregnancy, be sure to use some form of birth control. Research the many options available, and determine which one is best for you.

Infections can be passed during sex play from skin-to-skin contact or through the sharing of body fluids, such as blood, semen, pre-cum and vaginal fluids. Sexually active people can reduce their risk of infection during sex play by practicing safer sex.

Some people believe that condoms should be used every single time you engage in any sex play unless pregnancy is intended, while some feel that partners in a monogamous relationship should both be tested for STIs before engaging in sex play without a condom. There is a wide range of perspective, and while neither is right or wrong, it is a personal decision that is best for you.

Some sexually transmitted infections can be treated and cured with antibiotics. Others can be treated, but there is no cure, such as HIV (Human Immunodeficiency Virus), the virus that causes AIDS.

Communication is a must when talking about safer sex practices. Create a safe, COMFORTABLE environment for discussion, whether it's parents, children or partner, and this will breed confidence. Sexual health is too important, that is why it is so important to be comfortable with your sexuality and discussing safer sex and condom usage.

One of the big problems I have seen and heard since I started selling sex toys was with couples that don't talk about sex. This is probably what has driven me over the years and why I continue to educate and empower women and men about their own sexuality.

You need to be able to converse with your partner in every aspect of your relationship including sex, both in and out of the bedroom.

Understand the fear that surrounds the discussions about sex and sexuality. In addition to embarrassment, some people may have a fear of rejection, or fear of disclosing socially "inappropriate" sexual desires. While these fears are often justified since we also live in a culture of fast and harsh judgment, they make it very difficult for us to talk about sex honestly with the people around us. Give permission that it's okay to feel those feelings. Say something like "It's ok to be embarrassed or uncomfortable, I get embarrassed to" and you normalize it.

I had a customer once who told me how her partner would always "nibble" at her ear to signal to her that he wanted to have sex. She didn't explain how she knew this was the "signal" because he never told her so, but she HATED it. I asked her if she ever told him she didn't like that. Her response was, "I don't want to hurt his feelings".

Now, while I understand that she would like to spare him the rejection, if she doesn't tell him, he will keep on doing it, and if she hasn't grown to love it now, she probably never will. Besides, do you think your partner wants to do something they know you hate? Not in a healthy relationship they don't.

While still in the thick of it, suggest something that you do like instead of telling your partner that you don't like what they're doing. Your enthusiasm is much more exciting that your disapproval. Even though it is not your intent to criticize, you don't want it to be perceived as such.

Perhaps wait until any other time but the heat of the moment to kindly tell your partner, that you don't like that ear nibble as much as they do. Wouldn't it be funny if they hated it too, and only did it because they thought YOU liked it? How did that whole thing even start anyway, do you remember?

This is why it's so important to know your own body, what you like, and what you don't like. Remember, just as our bodies are individual and unique, so is what turns us on. Realizing what feels good is part of what makes sex play fun and enjoyable. And partners can only know what they like when they communicate that to each other, either verbally or by showing them with our body language.

If there is a new or different sexual activity that you want to try, suggest it to your partner. You may feel embarrassed, vulnerable, or even silly, but whatever your feelings are you should feel safe sharing your wants and desires with your partner. There are also things you can do to help the conversation go more smoothly.

Do not assume that your partner will think you are weird for suggesting a new sexual behavior. Often, these fears are worse than the reality and you'll never know until you ask.

Practice the conversation ahead of time. Predicting your partner's questions or concerns will help you feel more confident asking for what you want.

Ask in the sexiest way possible. If it's easier to write it down than to verbalize it face to face, go for it. That's a start. Maybe leave a sexy note on their pillow, in their car, or pack it in with their lunch. Again, you are only limited by your imagination.

Never pressure your partner into trying a sexual behavior that she or he is not comfortable with. It may take time to warm up to your ideas, so "no" could mean "not now". Don't perceive it to mean, "no way, not ever". Either way, just be patient and non-judgmental.

Ask your partner to share her or his desires. Maybe there is something your partner would like to try but hasn't had the nerve to bring up.

Do not believe that your partner is not attracted to you or does not care for you just because he or she says "no" to a behavior that you suggest. Remember, your partner is rejecting the behavior, not you.

Sex should never feel like an obligation or a chore. It should not feel like an inconvenience, duty or part of your martial responsibility. Always respect your partner's limits and boundaries about what he or she wants to do and does not want to do. Period.

It is normal to have concerns about a partner's reaction when proposing something new. But talking about what excites one another and what feels good and what is arousing can help sex partners have richer and more satisfying sex lives.

It also develops communication, trust, and openness in a relationship.

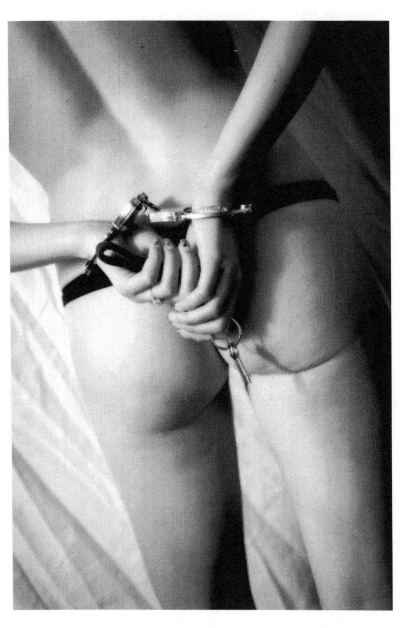

Photo by Studio1923.com

CHAPTER 6

Boundaries

You have the right & responsibility

Comfort and security with your sexuality begin with feeling safe. Safety, respect, consent, communication and ground rules are the standard components in setting boundaries for healthy sexual communication as well as mutually satisfying sex play.

You have the right and responsibility to protect yourself and your body. Only you can decide who you share your thoughts, your body, and your sexual experiences with, and no one has the right to touch you without your permission.

Sex partners need to practice good communication and be in agreement about shared sex play. Words, gestures, and actions are all ways that people can consent to sex. However, it is extremely important never to mistake your partner's intentions. Either player can stop at any time. If either person isn't feeling okay at any point they need to be able to pause everything and have their needs attended to.

We have the right and the responsibility to say no to, and/or stop sex play if we start to feel uncomfortable. Just as we need to be able to verbalize our sexual wants and desires by asking for what we want, being able to communicate what we don't want is just as important in any healthy relationship.

As previously stated in Chapter 5, always respect your partner's limits and boundaries about what they want and don't want. You have the right to have your limits and boundaries respected as well.

Without consent, sex can also have legal ramifications. Drugs and alcohol may impair an individual's ability to agree to sexual activity. Do not have sex with someone who is too drunk or too high to give consent.

It is also illegal for adults to engage in sexual behavior or sexually explicit discussions with minors. This includes online chats, emails and text messages. The age of consent varies from state to state.

You have the right and responsibility to protect yourself always. Make sure someone is old enough and sober enough to consent to sex before engaging in any sex play.

Talking about sex, sexuality, responsibility, ground rules and consent can be awkward because you are revealing yourself and that makes you vulnerable. Remember, good sexual communication, as well as good sex, means having a clear sense of personal boundaries. Without them, you may disclose more than you're comfortable with or even take more responsibility for the person you're talking to than you really should.

Developing boundaries isn't something that happens overnight. It is usually a practice of pushing the limits to get a sense of what you are comfortable with. It also allows a better understanding of what you may not be comfortable with. Good sexual communication should never feel like it crosses the line.

I do this on a daily basis. While I am a passionate believer that sex is not a dirty word, I understand not everyone shares my enthusiasm or conviction. While I am respectful that not everyone who asks me what I do for a living *really* wants to hear about how I empower others to have a fulfilling sex life, those barriers still need to come down. I, and other "sexperts" and pleasure peddlers like me, continue to chip away at those obstacles so that more men and women can and will enhance their sexual experiences, thus creating more satisfying relationships. It has been said that "Couples that play together, stay together".

I give permission to share without judgment something that is essential in any communication. Permission, ground rules, and boundaries apply to talking about sex as much as they apply to having it. We expose a part of ourselves when we initiate a new sexual conversation with anyone; but especially a new, long-term and/or committed partner. Since this can still make you feel ill at ease, you may bypass it completely. Keep the lines of communication open and two-way. It is necessary to keep a long-term sexual relationship thriving.

No one can be expected to talk honestly and openly unless they feel safe. Do you know what you need in order to feel safe? Do you know what your partner needs in order to feel safe? Define safety for yourself as well as your partner. If you agree on things like a judgment-free zone in order to communicate freely and easily, that becomes one of the ground rules. Some ground rules should be common sense and some are just common courtesy.

For example, if the conversation you're having is about experimenting with sexual fantasies or things you might want to experience together, remember to agree to be respectful of the differences in sexual interests. Remember, never belittle, shame, or laugh at a partner's sexual interests. This doesn't mean you're obligated to like them or try them, but if your partner takes the risk of revealing a sexual desire, consider that kind of exposure a compliment and be respectful, even if you want nothing to do with the actual proposal. Laying down ground rules is essential to creating a space that will feel safe.

If you decide to give it a go, remember that the same rules apply. No laughing at your partner for something they say or do. Avoid judgment. There is nothing wrong with having preferences, and you'll never be okay with everything someone wants to do, but everyone should learn to say no without putting someone down.

Respect is also essential when talking about sex. Even if you're just conversing casually with your girlfriends over drinks after work or at a gathering of several couples, respect the differences in sexual interests. If we make negative comments about a certain behavior that someone in the group takes great pleasure in, anal sex for example, it can create those feelings of shame we are trying to disassociate all together form sex.

Listen. Listen to your children, listen to your friends, and listen to your parents, too. If someone wants to talk to you, or needs to talk to you about sex, listen. Always listen to your partner. This is one the hardest ground rules to follow, but it is the most important. If someone wants to talk to you about sex, again, consider it a compliment that they feel safe talking to you, so listen without interrupting, and be respectful.

Understand your limits and learn how to withdraw from conversations or activities that make you feel uncomfortable. While others may feel safe confiding in you, there may come a time when conversations cross your personal boundaries. Know how to manage conversations that may be beyond your scope, and how to separate yourself if you need to.

Remember that if you're interrupting and talking over each other, neither one of you will feel like you've been heard. Agree to not interrupt and know that you'll both slip up, but when you do you'll apologize and try harder to listen and wait before responding.

A basic rule of good communication skills is to talk about yourself and your own feelings. Avoid telling the other person how they feel or what they think because in reality, you have no idea. A simple way to do this is try to start sentences with "I", as in *"I feel like this when you do that"*.

Relationships require compromise, but it doesn't mean we can't have our own thoughts, feelings and principles. Show each other enough respect for all differences without forcing either person to concede their beliefs. In the end, everyone has to compromise, but in the beginning everyone should be allowed to be heard.

Most people need to feel like what they say in a private conversation stays private. You will have to agree on the confines of your discussions (is it OK to talk to a best friend? A brother or sister?) But whatever restrictions you put on it, you have to respect those boundaries and keep it confidential.

In order to maintain the feeling of safety, everyone needs to feel like they can disengage at any time. This does not make it okay to storm out while your partner (or anyone else) is in the middle of a sentence, but agree that anyone, at any point, can ask for a time out, or to end the conversation if you begin to feel uncomfortable or unsafe. Agree to pick it up at a later point.

The same is true during sex play. Anyone can stop a scene at any time. Especially during fantasy sexual roleplay, which can be intense, and can bring up feelings that may be surprising, so it's important to remember that the point is to have fun, and enjoy each other. Again, if at any time either person feels uncomfortable, they can stop. Those needs must be met.

Whether you're talking about sex play or having sex play, the ground rules and boundaries are very similar. You have the right to feel safe and respected. If you can communicate your wants and desires, you can experiment and explore all sorts of possibilities.

You have the right and responsibility to set ground rules when experimenting with new sex play or sex acts. Participating in any type of sexual fantasy roleplay should incorporate the use of a safe word. This word should be established prior to sexual activity.

A safe word is a word that is usually irrelevant and strange in context of the sexual situation. Generally used in the BDSM community, it has migrated into all forms of foreplay and anal play. The safe word is agreed by the participating player to either modify or cease the activity.

This is so that either partner can say "stop" and "no" as part of their play as often as they want and use the safe word when they actually mean it. Sexual safe words could also be called sexual trust words and they're an especially good idea in any kind of sex play that is exploratory and/or new to any player.

Safe words should be ones that a participant isn't likely to use as part of their play. They can be complete code like APPLES (stop), CLEVELAND (slow down) and MARSHMALLOW (don't stop) or more obvious like "red", "yellow" and "green".

In the practice of Sado-masochism, a safe word is established and uttered by the recipient when he/she can no longer tolerate any more pain administered by the sadist during a session. It may also be used to indicate they need a "break" in the session.

No kind of sex should EVER be forced on anyone at any time...that's called RAPE (which is totally different than indulging in an agreed upon rape fetish) and the basic idea of safe words is to prevent rape from happening accidentally.

Ground rules are usually well established in non-monogamy and other interpersonal relationships in which an individual forms multiple and simultaneous sexual and/or romantic bonds. An open relationships is one in which the partners involved agree that they want to be together, but in which romantic or sexual relationships with additional people are accepted, permitted or tolerated

Boundaries are necessary no matter what type of sex play, activity or relationship you choose to partake in. You have the right to make your own choices, no matter how accepted they may or may not be, as part of expressing your sexuality.

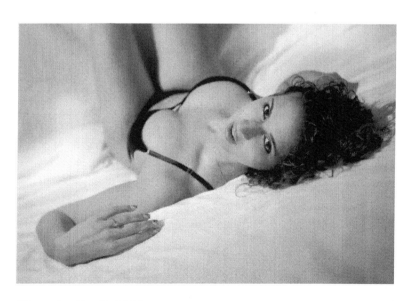

Photo by Studio1923.com

CHAPTER 7

Celebrate your sexuality out loud

Local to global

This is how I celebrate my sexuality.

I work in a field that makes tons of people feel uncomfortable. I do my best to be kind and treat everyone with understanding and to make them feel comfortable by normalizing what I do. After all, it is normal to me.

I listen to what people have to say, which is not always pleasant, courteous or favorable. I respect their opinions, and I try to have responses ready. I do not attempt to change anyone's mind; I just invite them to open it a bit.

One of the many lessons I have learned over the years is that some will embrace me and what I do and some will not. I used to take it personally and wondered why people would judge me so severely without knowing anything about me.

I believe in what I do. I believe in every product that I endorse and I believe that everyone has the right to enjoy and enhance their own sexual experiences with or without a partner. So what if some do not share my beliefs, because for every person that looks down on me for my profession, somewhere, someone is waiting for me and my message.

Sexual orientation and gender are fundamental parts of who we are. Whether we are female, male, or intersex and whether our gender is our biological, social, and legal status as men or women. Sexual orientation is the term used to describe whether a person feels sexual desire for people of the opposite gender, same gender, or both genders. The more we understand biological sex, gender, gender identity, and sexual orientation, the more we may understand and appreciate sexual diversity.

Everyone expresses their sexuality in a different way, and some we may be more aware and accepting of then others. And while there is still rejection over many sexuality issues in our society — including homophobia, sexism, and transphobia - fortunately many are brave, proud, and live out loud.

PRIDE is the concept that Lesbian, Gay, Bisexual and Transgender people should be proud of their sexual orientation and gender identity. The movement also supports that diversity is a gift and that sexual orientation and gender identity are inherent and cannot be intentionally altered. PRIDE events take place all over the world often with parades and festivals catering to and celebrating the LGBT communities.

The word PRIDE is used as an antonym for shame, which has been used to control and oppress Lesbian, Gay, Bisexual and Transgender persons throughout history. The use of the abbreviated "Gay Pride" and "Pride" expression have become mainstream and shortened expressions inclusive of all individuals in LGBT communities.

The most widely known symbol representing gay pride is perhaps the pride flag. The Rainbow flag is multi-colored and consists of stripes in the colors of the rainbow. The design is based on the traditional scheme of red, orange, yellow, green, blue and purple. The use of rainbow flags has a long tradition; they are displayed in many cultures around the world as a symbol of diversity and inclusiveness, of hope and of yearning.

~~~~~~~~~~~~~~~~~~~~

Sexual fantasy and/or role-playing is another form of expressing one's sexuality. It can include dressing up and acting out an erotic scene from a movie. It could also bring back steamy memories of the complicated and luscious roles taken on in the heat of passion. For many people sexual fantasy roleplay is something that intrigues them, but with some fear of judgment.

Once that apprehension passes, sexual fantasy and roleplay opens up a new world of sexual experiences. It is a magnificent way to liberate ourselves, temporarily, from the restrictions and responsibilities of our daily life and take on the role of someone else.

Fantasy is a significant part of sexual pleasure. Some sexual fantasies are momentary. For example, we might think for a few seconds about seeing an actor naked or about being gratified in a certain way. Other Sexual fantasies are longer. For example, we may remember a sexual encounter we have previously experienced while we self-serve or have sex play with others.

~~~~~~~~~~~~~~~~~

The Internet has opened up a whole other world of sexual expression. Cybersex, also called computer sex, Internet sex, netsex, mudsex, TinySex and, colloquially, cybering, is a virtual sex encounter in which two or more persons connect remotely via computer network and send each other sexually explicit messages describing a sexual experience. It is a form of sexual roleplay in which the participants may pretend they are having actual sex. In one form, this fantasy sex is accomplished by the participants describing their actions and responding to their chat partners in a mostly written form designed to stimulate their own sexual feelings and fantasies.

Cybersex may include real life masturbation. It can occur either within the context of an existing relationship, perhaps among partners who are geographically separated, or among individuals who have no prior knowledge of one another and meet in virtual spaces or cyberspaces.

The anonymity of such encounters can be good practice for verbalizing wants and desires and also add to the excitement. It is also a safe form of exploration, where there is no exchange of bodily fluids between the participants. In some contexts cybersex is enhanced by the use of a webcam to transmit real-time video of the partners.

~~~~~~~~~~~~~~~~~~~~~

Some sexual behaviors may be considered unconventional. **BDSM** is a gamut of erotic practice and expression involving the consensual use of restraint, intense sensory stimulation, and fantasy roleplay. The compound acronym, BDSM, is derived from the terms bondage and discipline (B&D or B/D), dominance and submission (D&S or D/s), and sadism and masochism (S&M or S/M).

BDSM includes an expansive range of activities, forms of interpersonal relationships, and distinct subcultures.

The fundamental principles for the exercise of BDSM require that it should be performed by responsible partners, of their own volition, in a safe way. Since the 1980s these basic principles have been condensed into the motto "Safe, sane and consensual", abbreviated as SSC, which means that everything is based on safe, sane and consenting behavior of all involved parties. This mutual consent makes a clear legal and ethical distinction between BDSM and crimes such as sexual assault or domestic violence.

Aside from the general advice related to safe sex, BDSM sessions often require a wider array of safety precautions than typical vanilla sex (sexual behavior without BDSM elements) such as the "safe" words we mentioned in chapter six.

~~~~~~~~~~~~~~~~~

People celebrate their sexuality when they choose a life partner or settle on a monogamous relationship. While the social norm has been through traditional matrimonial bonds, today scores of committed couples choose not to marry. Others may choose non-monogamy, or an open relationship with more than one partner, while some prefer a poly-amorous relationship.

An open relationship is where the people involved agree that they want to be together, but accept, allow or tolerate romantic or sexual relationships with additional people. This is a generalization of the concept of open marriage beyond marital relationships.

Open marriage typically refers to a marriage in which the partners consent that each may engage in extramarital sexual relationships, without being considered as infidelity or betrayal. There are many different styles of open marriage, with the partners having varying levels of input on their spouse's activities.

Couples in open marriages may favor different kinds of relationships outside the marriage. Couples who prefer relationships emphasizing love and emotional involvement have a polyamorous style of open marriage. Couples who prefer extramarital relationships emphasizing sexual gratification and recreational friendships have a swinging style of open marriage. These distinctions may depend on psychological factors such as sociosexuality and may contribute to the formation of separate Polyamory and swinging communities.

Polyamory is the practice or acceptance of having more than one intimate relationship at a time with the knowledge and consent of everyone involved. Polygamy is plural marriage and has been brought into the mainstream thanks to shows like HBO's "Big Love" and TLC's "Sister Wives".

Despite their distinctions, however, most open relationships' marriages share common issues: the lack of social acceptance, the need to maintain the health of their relationship and avoid neglect, and the need to manage jealous rivalry.

Many couples have clear negotiated rules. For example, there is to be no emotional attachment, partners must always use protection, relations are never to occur in the family bed/home, no illegitimate children, and/or must (or must not) know who the other person is, to name a few of the most common. Some open relationships are one sided, perhaps one partner may need more sexual gratification than the other, and is free to seek it out where he/she sees fit, all while maintaining a functional emotional relationship with their full-time partner.

While "open relationship" is sometimes used as a synonym for "polyamorous relationship", these terms are generally differentiated. The "open" in "open relationship" usually refers to the sexual aspect of a non-closed relationship, whereas "polyamory" refers to the extension of a relationship by allowing bonds to form (which may be sexual or otherwise) as additional long term relationships. However, there is enough overlap between the two concepts that "open relationship" is sometimes used as a catch-all substitute when speaking to people who may not be familiar with polyamory.

~~~~~~~~~~~~~~~~~

Not everyone expresses their sexuality so loud and proud, and that is okay. As long as everyone can begin to emerge from the black cloud of negativity, shame, guilt and myths and step into the sunlight of comfort with their sexuality, then we can continue to move forward and change our world.

Explore your own feelings around issues related to sexuality. Embrace those feelings as part of your own sexuality identity without fear or guilt. While there are still many other forms of expression when it comes to sexuality in 21st century America, know that there is no wrong choice, as long as it is your own.

I sell sex toys for a living. That's the short answer. It was not my lifelong dream since I was a young girl. I discovered Athena's Home Novelties when I was at a pretty comfortable place in my own life. It started out as a hobby, became a part-time job and evolved into a serious business. Through my own journey of self-discovery and self-improvement and empowerment, I have discovered that this is my life's purpose.

I educate women and men on how to have a more satisfying sex life. I empower people to take control of their sexual experiences, to try new things. I encourage people to ask me questions without fear or judgment and normalize every conversation. I believe that sex toys enhance a woman's ability to achieve orgasm and renew feelings of excitement in mature relationships. I teach everyone to embrace their sexuality and communicate with their partners in and out of the bedroom. Over the years I have received cards, letters and emails from people who have discovered through me that it is okay to have sex and enjoy it. This reminds me that my work is not only promising, but purposeful.

I lead a team of women and men, who do what I do, and each has graced my life with their presence and radiance, and I honor each one of them.

I have met others who sell sex toys for countless different reasons, and we encompass an undeniable unity in our diversity. We are women and men of every sexual orientation and marital status from nearly every ethnicity, economic class and social standing.

I have been introduced to famous authors, world renowned speakers and celebrities.

It has been on this journey that I've been able to give back a little of what has been given to me with several VDAY efforts across the country and the Athena's Cup to break a world record and end breast cancer.

I have a loving, passionate relationship with my husband. I am a Goddess that is confident, powerful and comfortable with my own sexuality.

And I have done my best to create the culture of trust, safety and comfort that encourages open and honest conversations with my own daughters about sex and sexuality.

THAT is how I celebrate MY sexuality.

About the Author

Jenifer Bartoszek is a Sexual Health Examiner, a Certified Sex Educator, a Certified Dream Coach™, and a Goddess with Athena's Home Novelties, one of the country's premier adult novelty companies. Since 2004, and with a style that's witty, tasteful and fun, she has entertained and educated thousands. Today, Jenifer is still doing parties, and already thinking about her next book. She resides with her husband John and three daughters. For more information, please visit www.JeniferBartoszek.com

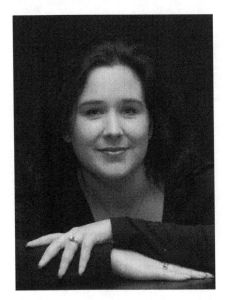

Photo by K. Gibson of EKG-Photography.com

Made in the USA
Charleston, SC
23 December 2011